YOUR KNOWLEDGE HAS VALUE

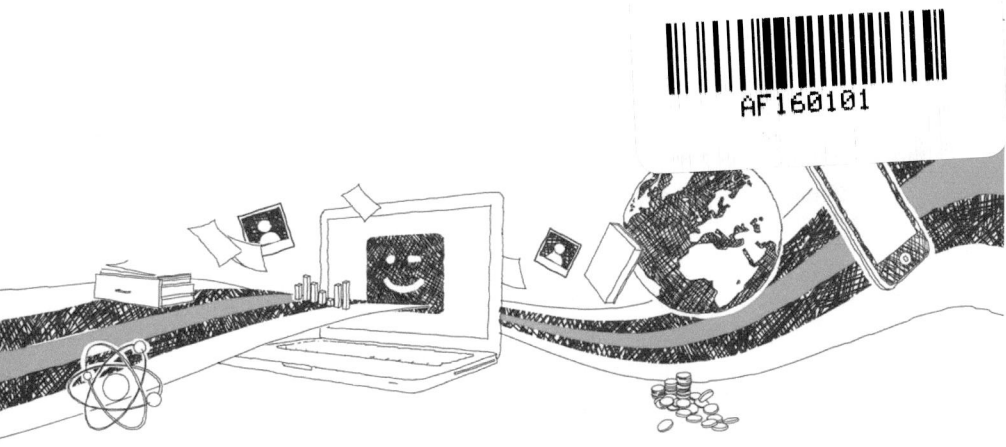

- We will publish your bachelor's and master's thesis, essays and papers

- Your own eBook and book - sold worldwide in all relevant shops

- Earn money with each sale

Upload your text at www.GRIN.com and publish for free

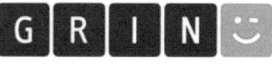

Bibliographic information published by the German National Library:

The German National Library lists this publication in the National Bibliography; detailed bibliographic data are available on the Internet at http://dnb.dnb.de .

This book is copyright material and must not be copied, reproduced, transferred, distributed, leased, licensed or publicly performed or used in any way except as specifically permitted in writing by the publishers, as allowed under the terms and conditions under which it was purchased or as strictly permitted by applicable copyright law. Any unauthorized distribution or use of this text may be a direct infringement of the author s and publisher s rights and those responsible may be liable in law accordingly.

Imprint:

Copyright © 2017 GRIN Verlag, Open Publishing GmbH
Print and binding: Books on Demand GmbH, Norderstedt Germany
ISBN: 9783668574113

This book at GRIN:

http://www.grin.com/en/e-book/380372/active-participation-of-male-in-family-planning

Rahima Begum, Sabina Islam, Samiha Noor Choudhury

Active Participation of Male in Family Planning

GRIN Publishing

GRIN - Your knowledge has value

Since its foundation in 1998, GRIN has specialized in publishing academic texts by students, college teachers and other academics as e-book and printed book. The website www.grin.com is an ideal platform for presenting term papers, final papers, scientific essays, dissertations and specialist books.

Visit us on the internet:

http://www.grin.com/

http://www.facebook.com/grincom

http://www.twitter.com/grin_com

ACTIVE PARTICIPATION OF MALE IN FAMILY PLANNING

Musa. Rahima Begum
Ph.D Research Fellow, Statistics Department, Shahjalal University of Science and Technology, Sylhet

Dr. Sabina Islam
Professor, Department of Statistics, Shahjalal University of Science and Technology, Sylhet

&

Samiha Noor Choudhury
Research Student, Statistics Department, Shahjalal University of Science and Technology, Sylhet

Abstract

Men are partners in reproduction and sexuality. It is therefore required that both men and women equally share satisfying sexual lives and the burden of preventing diseases and health complications. This paper studies the status of male active participants in family planning in Bangladesh and further explores the associated determinants. The study makes use of Bangladesh Demographic Health Survey, 2007 data (BDHS-2007). Bivariate analysis shows that age of the respondent, age of the partner, family type, respondent's desire for more children, partners' desire for more children, discuss FP with partner, education of the respondent, education of the partner and division are significantly associated with active participation of male in family planning. Logistic regression analysis identifies four significant determinants of active participation of male in family planning which are age of the respondent, age of the partner, education of the partner and discuss family planning with partner.

Key words: Male Participation, Family Planning

1. INTRODUCTION   2

2. DATA AND METHODOLOGY   3

3. RESULTS   3
   3.1 Differentials in active participation of male in family planning   4
   3.2 Determinants of the active participation of male in FP   7

4. DISCUSSION AND CONCLUSION   8

REFERENCES   10

1. INTRODUCTION

Male's involvement in family planning is defined as the men's decision regarding reproductive health issues viz., reproductive rights of women, fertility and its control through direct participation in family planning. Both male and female involvement on fertility and reproductive health was the key message in 1994 International Conference on Population and Development and Fourth World Conference (1995) on Women. It is argued that men are partners in reproduction and sexuality, and therefore it is logical that they equally share satisfying sexual lives and the burden of preventing diseases and health complications (Green et al.,1995). A number of researchers have identified that men are directly responsible for preventing pregnancy through coital-dependent methods such as condoms, withdrawal and periodic abstinence (Greene and Biddlecom, 2000). Historically, the traditional method withdrawal (coitus interrupts) has been used as a contraceptive method since ancient time (PA1, 1991). And use of condom dates back to 400 years (Ross and Frankenberg, 1993). Worldwide, one-third of the eligible couples using family planning rely on methods (vasectomy, condom, withdrawal and periodic abstinence) which require full male co-operation (Hossain, 2003). Men's acceptance of vasectomy and condoms were found numerous, reflecting the public health problem of sexually transmitted diseases (Bertrand et al.1989; Grady et al.,1993; Greene and Biddlecom, 2000; Ringheim, 1993; Ross and Huber, 1983). Kondel and Pramualratana (1996) conducted a study in Thailand and revealed that while men may think condom use is good in general; their views of actually using condom in sexual relation with spouses may be negative because of the association between condoms and promiscuity, disease and commercial sex. Studies in Uganda and Tanzania reveals little support among men for condom use within marriage (Blance et al., 1996; Pool et al., 1996).

By virtue of tradition and associated social factors, men in China have an active influence upon decisions about which method of contraception will be used in the family. Yunnan and Jilin provinces in 1992 suggested that, in Sichuan province 34 percent of all contraceptive acceptors relied upon male sterilization and 4 percent upon condom (Anonymous, 1995). Low level of male involvement in use of contraceptives is influenced by a misconception about family planning (Akafuah and Sossou, 2008). One of the main findings of this study was that increasing people's knowledge, changing attitudes, practices of family planning and reproductive decision-making can be influenced by exposure to mass-media education. Demographic factors, religion, education, types of marital relationship can also have positive impact in this regard. Another finding of the study is that the people's lack of knowledge causes socio-cultural misconceptions. Lack of education is the reason cited for not using various family planning methods (Akafuah and Sossou, 2008).

Bangladesh spousal communication is poor and this often makes it difficult for men to understand the reproductive health problems of women. Prevailing culture and myth do not allow men to visit health facilities with their wives. Husbands do not feel comfortable taking their wives to a health facility because they do not like to discuss sexual and reproductive health issues with the service providers (Kabir and Shahjahan 2007).

Men can actively participate in family planning by using any methods viz. condom, male sterilization, periodic abstinence and withdrawal. According to BDHS 2007 the rate of condom user, male sterilization, withdrawal and periodic abstinence are 4.5 percent, 0.7 percent, 2.9 percent and 4.9 percent respectively. Men active participation in family planning is now a growing substance of study. The participation of male in contraception is widely varies with the variation in some socio-economic and demographic characteristic Ghafur and Tehmina, 2005, Islam et el 2005; Olawepo and Oledare, 2006). Therefore this study makes an attempt to find the differential of male active participation in family planning and try to identify the influencing factors that contribute in male participation in family planning activities in Bangladesh.

2. DATA AND METHODOLOGY

The study utilized the matched sample of 3771 husbands with their wives who have participated in the BDHS 2007. The BDHS-2007 survey was conducted under the authority of the National Institute for Population Research and Training (NIPORT) of the Ministry of Health and Family Welfare. Mitra and Associates executed the survey with the technical assistance from ORC Macro and financial support from USAID (NIPORT *et al.*, 2005). The variables that are significantly associated with the active participation examined using bivariate analyses are further explored using binary logistic regression techniques. The dependent variable in the logistic regression analysis is 'Active participation of male'. The variable takes the value 'one' if respondents actively participating in family planning by using any of the method viz, condom, male sterilization, withdrawal and periodic abstinence. And 'zero' otherwise. The study has dealt with a large number of explanatory variables such as age of the respondent, age of the partner, respondent's age at first marriage, marital duration, ideal number of boys, ideal number of girls, ideal number of children, family type, ideal family size, number of living children, respondent's desire for more children, partner's desire for more children, discuss FP with partner, respondent approves FP, current working status of partner, religion, education of the respondent, respondent's occupation, place of residence and exposure to mass media.

3. RESULTS

The participation of male in Family planning method is very low in Bangladesh. Though contraceptive prevalence rate is high (55.8 %) in Bangladesh (BDHS, 2007) but by utilizing the BDHS, 2007 data we find that only ten percentage male actively participate in family planning in Bangladesh (Table 1). Fears among men about losing control; lack of political commitment; policy barriers (strict eligibility criteria for vasectomy); provider bias (programs oriented toward women); and inadequate information may lag behind men from family planning (Green *et. al.*, 1995). Partner support is a significant predictor of the likelihood that women will attempt to use a contraceptive method (Burwell, 1996; Green, 1994). Providing men with information and involving them in counseling sessions can help them supportive of contraceptive use and more aware of the concept of sharing decision making (Wells, 1997).

Table 1: Active Participation of Male in FP: BDHS 2007

Actively Participate	Number of respondents	Percentage
Yes	387	10.26
No	3384	89.73
Total	3771	

3.1 Differentials in active participation of male in family planning

Differentials in active participation of male in family planning are examined here in order to find the significant factors, which influence contraceptive behaviour. Our study finds active participation of male has significant association with age of the respondent and age of partner. We observed that active participation is the lowest among males whose age above 45 years (8.4 %) and as the partners age increase the participation of male also increases (Table 2). The participation does not associated with respondent's age at first marriage, marital duration, ideal number of boys, ideal number of girls, ideal number of children, ideal family size, number of living children, respondent approves FP, current use of contraceptives, religion, education of the respondent, respondent's occupation, place of residence and exposure to mass media.

Family type significantly associated with active participation of male in family planning. It is found that active participation is higher (10.8%) in nuclear family than in extended family (8.5%). Higher participation is viewed who are undecided and partners want no more children. Among those who actively participated in FP 16% of them discuss FP with partner. Though respondent education does not significantly associated but with the increase in the level of partners education respondents participation increase (Table3.2).

Active participation differs significantly within the regions. The rate of participation is the highest in Chittagong division (13.6 percent). Sylhet appeared as low performing region of contraceptive use in various studies (Kamal, 2008; Khan and Raeside, 1998; Mannan and Beaujot, 2006) but the rate of male active participation in Sylhet region is higher (10.0%) than Dhaka (7.5%) and Khulna (6.6%) (Table 2)

Table 2: Distribution of Active Participation of Male in FP According to Background Characteristics: BDHS 2007

| Background characteristics | Active participation | | Total | Chi-square (χ^2) |
	Yes	No		
Age of the respondent				
<35	11.0 (153)	89.0 (1234)	36.8(1387)	
35-45	11.0 (140)	89.0 (1131)	33.7(1271)	5.66**
≥45	8.4 (94)	91.6 (1019)	29.5(1113)	
Age of the partner				
<25	7.5 (93)	92.5 (1147)	32.9(1240)	
25-35	9.9 (127)	90.1 (1151)	33.9(1278)	23.21***
≥35	13.3 (167)	86.7 (1086)	33.2(1253)	
Respondent's age at first marriage				
<19	8.1 (41)	91.9 (466)	13.4(507)	
19-22	9.2 (80)	90.8 (789)	23.0(869)	7.57
22-25	10.2 (90)	89.8 (789)	23.3(879)	

25-28	12.3 (96)	87.7 (682)	20.6(778)	
≥28	10.8 (80)	89.2 (658)	19.6(738)	
Marital duration				
<5	11.3 (89)	88.7 (671)	20.2(760)	
5-10	10.9 (78)	89.1 (639)	19.0(717)	
10-15	11.7 (68)	88.3 (536)	16.0(604)	8.11
15-20	8.7 (49)	91.3 (517)	15.0(566)	
20-25	10.8 (51)	89.2 (421)	12.5(472)	
≥25	8.0 (52)	92.0 (600)	17.3(652)	
Ideal no of boys				
0	9.7 (108)	90.3 (1011)	31.0(1119)	
1	10.6 (194)	89.4 (1629)	50.5(1823)	1.17
2+	9.4 (63)	90.6 (605)	18.5(668)	
Ideal no of girls				
0	9.6 (117)	90.4 (1105)	33.9(1222)	
1	10.6 (228)	89.4 (1923)	59.6(21510	1.68
2+	8.4 (20)	91.6 (217)	6.6(237)	
Ideal no of children				
0	10.4 (261)	89.6 (2252)	69.6(2513)	
1	8.9 (14)	91.1 (144)	4.4(158)	
2	9.5 (71)	90.5 (673)	20.6(744)	1.49
3	8.7 (13)	91.3 (136)	4.1(149)	
≥4	13.0 (6)	87.0 (40)	1.3(46)	
Family type				
Nuclear	10.8 (316)	89.2 (2623)	77.9(2939)	3.47**
Extended	8.5 (71)	91.5 (761)	22.1(832)	
Ideal family size				
Small family	10.6 (206)	89.4 (1857)	54.7(2063)	0.38
Large family	10.0 (181)	90.0 (1527)	45.3(1708)	
Number of living children				
0	7.5 (32)	92.5 (392)	11.2(424)	
1-2	10.6 (174)	89.4 (1465)	43.5(1639)	4.22
3-4	10.9 (126)	89.1 (1028)	30.6(1154)	
5+	9.9 (55)	90.1 (499)	14.7((554)	
Respondent's desire for more children				
Wants no more	10.3 (241)	89.7 (2137)	65.2(2378)	
Wants another	10.1 (117)	89.9 (1039)	31.7(1156)	5.67**
Undecided	17.1 (19)	82.9 (92)	3.0(111)	
Partner's desire for more children				
Wants no more	12.7 (257)	87.3 (1772)	61.8(2029)	
Wants another	9.1 (110)	90.9 (1105)	37.0(1215)	12.93***
Undecided	2.6 (1)	97.4 (38)	1.2(39)	
Discuss FP with partner				
No	7.0 (141)	93.0 (1880)	57.3(2021)	76.31***
Yes	16.3 (245)	83.7 (1262)	42.7(1507)	
Respondent approves FP				
No	8.4 (22)	91.6 (241)	7.4(263)	1.17
Yes	10.5 (344)	89.5 (2938)	92.6(3282)	

Current working status of partner				
Working	10.2 (87)	89.8 (763)	22.4(850)	0.00
Not working	10.2 (299)	89.8 (2619)	77.4(2918)	
Religion				
Muslim	10.2 (345)	89.8 (3035)	89.6(3380)	0.11
Non Muslim	10.7 (42)	89.3 (349)	10.4(391)	

Table 2(Continued): Distribution of Active Participation of Male in FP According to Background Characteristics: BDHS 2007

Background characteristics	Active participation		Total	Chi-square (χ^2)
	Yes	No		
Education of the respondent				
No education	10.4 (114)	89.6 (978)	29.0(1092)	
Primary	10.7 (129)	89.3 (1076)	32.0(1205)	1.14
Secondary	10.2 (96)	89.8 (843)	25.0(944)	
Higher	9.1 (48)	90.9 (482)	14.1(530)	
Education of the partner				
No education	6.5 (70)	93.5 (1002)	28.4(1072)	
Primary	8.7 (106)	91.3 (1117)	32.4(1223)	89.74***
Secondary	11.8 (141)	88.2 (1056)	31.8(1197)	
Higher	25.2 (70)	74.8 (208)	7.4(278)	
Respondent's occupation				
Land owner, farmer	9.7 (83)	90.3 (773)	22.7(8560)	
Laborer	10.8 (173)	89.2 (1429)	42.5(1602)	
Professional	11.8 (25)	88.2 (187)	24.1(212)	2.59
Business	10.0 (91)	90.0 (817)	5.6(908)	
Others	7.9 (15)	92.1(176)	1.1(191)	
Division				
Barisal	12.6 (62)	87.4 (429)	13.0(491)	
Chittagong	13.6 (83)	86.4 (526)	16.1(609)	
Dhaka	7.5 (57)	92.5 (702)	20.1(759)	28.46***
Khulna	6.6 (41)	93.4 (583)	16.5(624)	
Rajshahi	12.0 (94)	88.0 (692)	20.8(786)	
Sylhet	10.0 (50)	90.0 (452)	13.3(502)	
Place of residence				
Urban	9.7 (140)	90.3 (1303)	38.3(1443)	0.79
Rural	10.6 (247)	89.4 (2081)	61.7(2328)	
Exposure to mass media				
Yes	10.4 (343)	89.6 (2940)	87.1(3283)	0.95
No	9.0 (44)	91.0 (444)	12.9(488)	

3.2 Determinants of the active participation of male in FP

The variable those are found to have significant association with male active participation in FP are further considered as independent variables in logistic regression model to see their combined effect. Table 3 shows that only the variables age of the respondent, age of partner, discuss FP with partner, and education of the partner are the determinants of the active participation of male in FP.

Result of logistic regression shows that active participation is 0.695 times lower among the husbands aged 45 or above than reference group after controlling the effect of other variables. Males whose partners' age above 35 are 4.017 times more likely to actively participate in FP compared to those whose age is less than 25 (Table 3).

Usually husbands who discuss family planning with their wives are more likely to use male methods (Islam et al, 2010; Agha, 2009). Table 3 shows that discussion about family planning with partner has a significant effect on active participation of male in family planning. Husbands who discuss family planning with their partners are 3.0 times more likely to actively participate in family planning than the husbands who do not discuss family planning with their partners. There exists a positive relation between partner's level of education and the active participation. With the increase in level of partner's education the likelihood of active participation also increases. The odds ratio of active participation are found 1.35, 2.3, and 5.1 of the respondent whose partners level of education are primary, secondary and higher respectively.

Table 3: Logistic regression analysis of Active Participation on some selected demographic, socio-economic factors: BDHS 2007

Characteristics	Active participation				95% C.I for Exp(B)	
	coefficient (β)	S .E(β)	Wald statistics	Odds ratio Exp(B)	Lower	Upper
Age of the respondent						
≤34®	----	----	5.817	1.000	----	----
35-44	-0.020	0.148	0.018	0.981	0.734	1.311
45+	-0.364**	0.174	4.400	0.695	0.494	0.976
Age of partner						
<25®	----	----	60.785	1.000	----	----
25-35	0.436**	0.176	6.132	1.547	1.095	2.185
≥35	1.390***	0.197	49.570	4.017	2.727	5.915
Family type						
Nuclear®	----	----	----	1.000	----	----
Extended	-0.085	0.165	0.263	0.919	0.664	1.270
Respondent desire additional child						
Wants no more®	----	----	3.882	1.000	----	----
Wants another	-0.162	0.150	1.172	0.850	0.634	1.140
Undecided	0.426	0.307	1.930	1.531	0.839	2.793
Partner's desire for more children						
Wants no more®	----	----	1.404	1.000	----	----
Wants another	-0.850	0.634	1.140	0.960	0.697	1.322
Undecided	1.531	0.839	2.793	0.298	0.039	2.250

Discuss FP with partner						
No®						
Yes	1.101***	0.127	75.668	3.007	2.347	3.854
Education of the partner						
No education®	----	----	69.326	1.000	----	----
Primary	0.303*	0.179	2.850	1.354	0.952	1.925
Secondary	0.828***	0.177	21.789	2.288	1.616	3.238
Higher	1.628***	0.214	58.161	5.096	3.353	7.743
Division						
Sylhet ®	----	----	14.013	1.000	----	----
Chittagong	0.215	0.222	0.935	1.240	0.802	1.918
Dhaka	0.222	0.212	1.096	1.248	0.824	1.890
Khulna	-0.316	0.220	2.058	0.729	0.473	1.123
Rajshahi	-0.322	0.236	1.868	0.724	0.456	1.150
Barisal	0.134	0.205	0.425	1.143	0.765	1.707
Constant	-3.698***	0.308	144.168	0.025	----	----

® Represent reference category;   *** P<0.01; ** P<0.05; * <0.1

4. DISCUSSION AND CONCLUSION

Reproductive health is a state of complete physical, mental and social wellbeing and not merely the absence of disease or infirmity, in all matters relating to the reproductive system and to its functions and process. Reproductive health therefore implies that people are able to have satisfying and save sex life and that they have the capability to reproduce and the freedom to decide if, when, and how often to do so. Implicit to this last condition are the right of men and women to be informed and to have access to safe, effective, affordable and acceptable methods of their choice, as well as other methods of their choice for regulation of fertility which are not against the law, and the right of access to appropriate health care services that will enable women to go safety through pregnancy and childbirth and provide couples with the best chance for having healthy infant (UN, 1995). It is evident from the definition above that both men and women should have equal rights in fulfilling their reproductive needs. One of the programs implemented by the government in each country participating in the ICPD to ensure the reproductive health of its people is family planning which is defined as a program purposed to help couples or individuals reach their reproductive goals. These goals include: preventing unwanted pregnancies; decreasing high risk pregnancies; morbidity and mortality; and making family planning services that are qualified, affordable, acceptable, and accessible for all society members (BKKBN, 2004).

Male involvement in family planning and use of male methods were associated with the fertility decline and resulted in long term benefits for women. Individual motivation rather than choice of methods was more important for positive male participation in family planning (Karra et al, 1997). Helzner (1996) mentioned that men's active participation in family planning could raise the use of male contraceptive methods (condom and vasectomy), or male dependent traditional methods (withdrawal and abstinence). Men also could support their wives in using female contraceptive methods (IUD, pill, implant, and injections). According to Greene and Biddlecom (2000), the inclusion of men in the demographic studies of reproduction has been justified; because there was an assertion that men inhibit women who want to use contraception.

Studies from several nations have shown that reproductive health programs are likely to be more effective for women when men are actively involved (Drennan, 1998). There is evidence that a husband's disapproval leads to reduction in contraception (Bongaarts and Bruce, 1995; Kamal, 2000). Various studies have shown that providing men with information and involving them in counseling sessions can help them to be more supportive of contraceptive use, and more aware of the concept of sharing decision making (Wells, 1997). Terefe and Larson reported a study in Ethiopia where couples receiving husband–wife counseling showed an increase in contraceptive use after 1 year, compared to women who were counseled alone (Terefe and Larson, 1993).

In Bangladesh Kamal (2000) evaluated the effect of the woman's perception of her husband's approval of family planning on her current and future use of modern contraception, after controlling for selected socioeconomic and demographic factors and shows that most husbands support family planning, contraceptive use among those whose husbands do not approve of family planning is much lower. Schuler *et al.*, (1995) have found that women in Bangladesh were dependent on their husband's decisions in family planning and reproductive health.

Sabu and Peter (2005) found that about 85 percent husbands approved FP and about 11 percent husbands disapproved it. 50 percent of the couples had not discussed family planning matters among themselves. About 65 percent husbands were using contraceptives. 6.5 percent husbands were using condom. The percentage of withdrawal and male sterilization were 2.4 and 0.6 percents respectively.

The study examined the active participation of male in family planning. It revealed that the active participation of male in family planning is very low in Bangladesh. Out of 3771 married men only 10.26 percent husbands actively participated in family planning by using the male methods; condoms, male sterilization, periodic abstinence and withdrawal. The reasons of low performance may the lack of variety of male methods and the lower patronage of family planning services towards male in Bangladesh. It is urgently required to inspire men to strongly involve with the contraception and reproductive decision making. Along with various significant factors partners education and discussion of FP with their wives play vital role in active participation of male family planning methods Educational programme that encourage men and women to assume more responsibility in family planning, birth control, preventing unwanted births can improve male participation. Cultural programs may also take to encourage men to family planning activities.

REFERENCES

Akafuah, R. A. & Marie-Antonio Sossou (2008), "Attitude towards and Use of Knowledge about Family Planning among Ghanaian Men". *International Journal of Men's Health* 7 (2): 109-120.

Agha, Sohail, 2009 "Intentions to Use Contraceptive in Pakistan: Implication for Behaviour Change Campaigns",

Anonymous. (1995), "Who holds up half of heaven? Male involvement in family planning". Responses to ICPD. *China Population Today* 12(2):9-11.

Balaiah, D. (1999), "Contraceptive Knowledge, Attitude and Practices of Men in Rural Maharashtra". *Advances in Contraception* 15 (3): 217-234.

BDHS (2007), "Bangladesh Demographic and Health Survey", National Institute of Population Research and training (NIPORT), Dhaka Bangladesh. www.measuredhs.com/pubs/pdf/FR207/FR207[April-10-2009].pdf

Bertland, Jane T. et al. (1989),"Attitudes towards voluntary surgical contraception in four districts of Kenya", *Studies in Family Planning* 20(5): 281-288.

BKKBN (2004), "Laporan Hasil Analisis Lanjut Data SM- PFA 2002-2003": Hubungan Beberapa Faktor dengan Partisipasi Pria dalam ber-KB dan Kesehatan Reproduksi di Propinsi Jawa Tengah dan Jawa Timur, Jakarta.

Blance, Ann K. et al. (1996), "Negotiating Reproductive Outcomes in Uganda', Calverton MD: *Macro International Inc. And Institute of Statistics and Applied Economics* (Uganda).

Bongaarts J and Bruce J (1995), "The causes of unmet need for contraception and the social content of services", *Studies in Family Planning,* 26(2):57–75.

Burwell, L.C., Hoover, D.D. and Kouzis, D.K.A. (1996), "Stages of change for condom use: the influence of partner type, relationship and pregnancy factors", *Family Planning Perspectives*, 28, 101–109.

Drennan, M. (1998). "Reproductive health: new perspectives on men's participation". Population Reports, Series J. N0-46. Baltimore, John Hopkins School of Public Health, *Population Information Program*

Ghafur, Tehmena (2005), "Male Invoelvement in Bangladesh's Reproductive Health Programme: A Status Report'' Population Review, Volume 44, Numer2, 2005

Grady, William R., Daniel H. Klepinger, John O.G. Billy, and Koray Tanfer (1993), "Condom Characteristics: The perceptions and Preferences of men in the United States", Family Planning Perspective 25(2): 67-73.

Green, C. P., Cohen, S. I. and Ghouayel, H. B. (1995). "Male Involvement in Reproductive Health, including Family Planning and Sexual Health". *Technical Report*, 28, UNFPA.

Green, C.P. (1994), "Male involvement in reproductive health and family planning",*UNFPA MIRH, Programme Advisory Note*.Technical Paper.

Green, M.E., A.E. Biddlecom,(2000), "Absent and Problematic Men; Demographic Accounts Of Male Reproductive Roles", *Population and Development Review* 26(1); pp.81-115

Helzner, JF (1996), "Men's Involvement in Family Planning", *Reproductive Health Matters*, No.7, May, pp.146-154.

Islam, M.A.;Sabu S, Padmas and Peter W.F. Smith(2005), "Degree and Determinants of Men's Contraceptive Knowledge in Bangladesh

Islam, M.A., Padmadas, S.S. and Smith, P.W.F. (2010) Understanding family planning communication between husbands and wives: a multilevel analysis of wives' responses from the Bangladesh DHS. Genus (in press)

Kabir, M. & Shahjahan M. (2007), "Why Males in Bangladesh Do Not Participate in Reproductive Health: Lessons Learned from Focus Group Discussions", *International Quarterly of Community Health Education*, Vol.26 (1): 45 - 59.

Kamal, N. (2000), "The influence of husbands on contraceptive use by Bangladeshi women". *Health Policy and Planning*, 15, 43–51.

Kamal, N. (2008), "Women's Autonomy and Uptake of Contraception in Bangladesh", *Centre for Health, Population and Development (CHPD), IUB*, Working Paper-16.

Khan H.T.A and Raeside (1998). "The determinants of first and subsequent births in urban and rural areas of Bangladesh", Asia Pacific Population Jounal, 13(2),pp.39-72

Karra, Mihira V. Nancy N. Stark and Joyce Wolf.(1997), "Male involvement in family planning; A case study spanning five generations of a South Indian Family", *Studies in Family Planning* 28(1);24-34

Kondel, J and A. Pramualratana (1996), "Prospects for increases condom use within marriage in Thailand", *International Family Planning Perspectives* 22(3): 97-102.

Mannan, H. R. and Beaujot, R. (2006), "Readiness , Willingness and Ability to Use Contraception in Bangladesh ". *Asia Pacific Population Journal,* vol. 2, No 1, April 2006.

NIPORT (2005), "National Institute of Population Research and Training, Mitra and Associates and Macro International, "Bangladesh Demographic and Health Survey- 2004", National Institute of Population, Research and Training Mitra and Associates and Maryland: Macro International, Dhaka, Bangladesh.

Olawepo R.A and Okedare E.A. (2006), "Men's Attitudes Towards Family Planning in a Traditional Urban Centre: An Example from Ilorin, Nigeria" *Journal of Social Science*, 13(2): 83-90.

PAI (1991) Population Action International. *"A Guide to Methods of Birth Control"*. Briefing Paper No. 25, Washington, D.C: PAI.

Pool, R., M. Maswe, J. T. Boerma, and S. Nnko (1996), "The price of promiscuity: why urban males in Tanzania are changing their sexual behavior", *Health Transition Review* 6: 203-222

Ringheim, Karin, (1993), "Factors that determine prevalence of use of contraceptive methods for men", Studies in Family planning 24(2): 87-99.

Ross, J. A. and Frankenberg, (1993) "Findings from Two Decades of Family Planning and Sexual Health" The Population council, New York, *International Family Planning Perspectives*, P-175.

Ross, John A. and Douglas H. Huber (1983), "Acceptance and prevalence of vasectomy in developing countries", *Studies in Family Planning* 14(3): 67-73.

Sabu S.;Islam .M.A. Padmadas and Peter W.F. (2005), "Men and family planning in Bangladesh: a multilevel approach using DHS data" International Population Conference, Tours (France), 18-23 Session 166: Male sexuality and contraception.

Schuler, SR, Hashemi, SM, Jenkins AH (1995), "Bangladesh's Family PlanningSuccess Story: A Gender Perspective", *International Family PlanningPerspectives*, Vol.21, No.4, December, pp.132-166.

Terefe, A. and Larson, C.P. (1993), "Modern contraception use in Ethiopia: does involving husbands make a difference?", *American Journal of Public Health,* 83, 1567–1576.

UN (1995), *"Report on the International Conference on Population and Development"*, United Nation Publication, New York.

Wells, E. (1997), "Involving men in reproductive health". Outlook, 14(3), 1–8.

YOUR KNOWLEDGE HAS VALUE

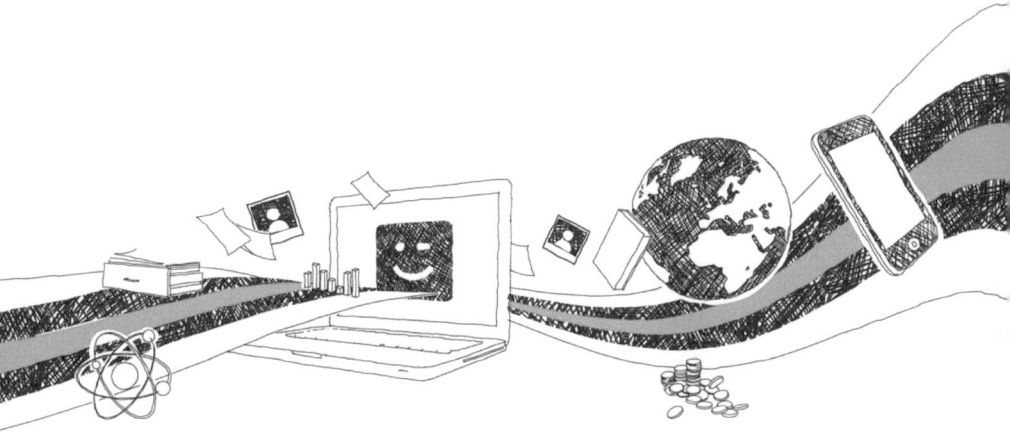

- We will publish your bachelor's and master's thesis, essays and papers

- Your own eBook and book - sold worldwide in all relevant shops

- Earn money with each sale

Upload your text at www.GRIN.com
and publish for free

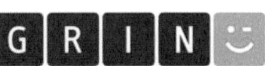